My Mom Has Gastroparesis

Timothy Thomas

AuthorHouse™
1663 Liberty Drive
Bloomington, IN 47403
www.authorhouse.com
Phone: 1 (800) 839–8640

Published by AuthorHouse 03/16/2015

ISBN: 978–1–4969–7483–9 (sc)
ISBN: 978–1–4969–7484–6 (e)

Library of Congress Control Number: 2015903652

Print information available on the last page.

authorHOUSE®

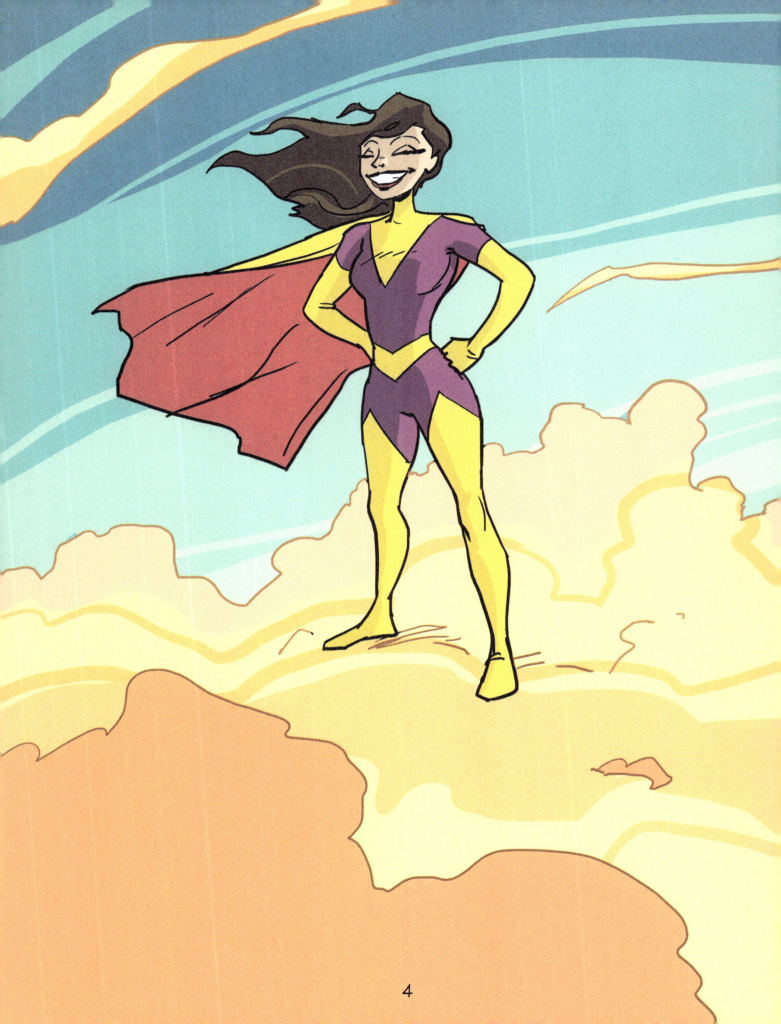

This is my mom. She is like any other mom. She loves me, takes care of me and is always there when I need her. Like a super hero.

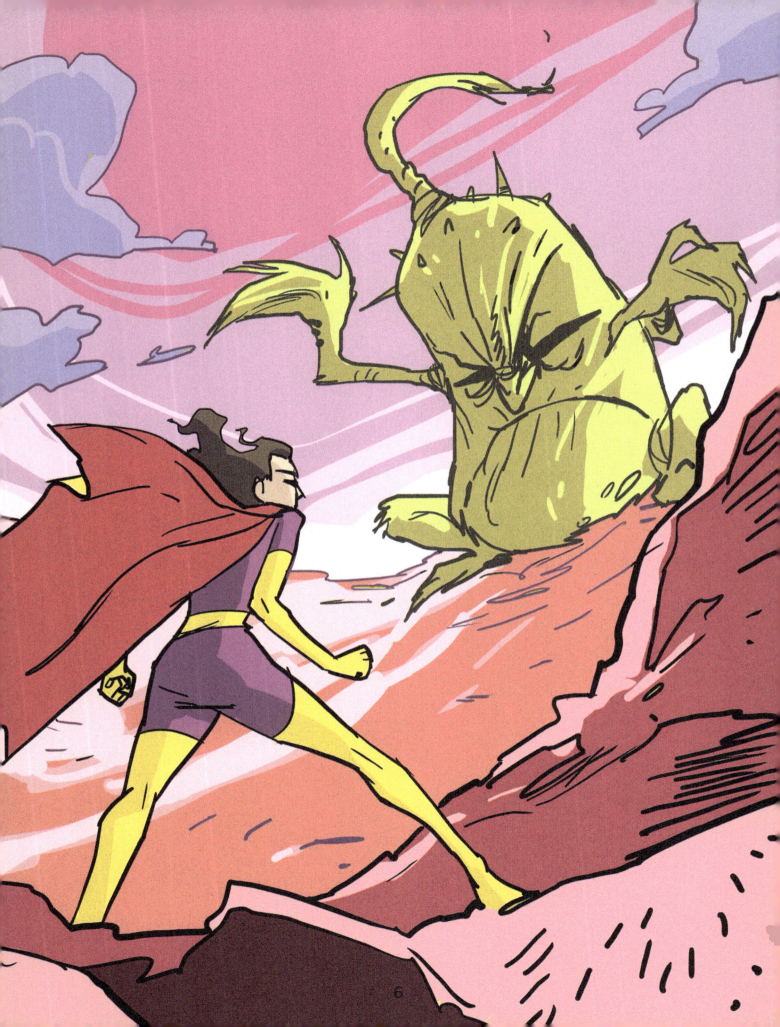

Like any superhero, My mom has her weakness like Kryptonite for Superman. My mom has something called Gastroparesis. It's called GP because Gastroparesis is too long and too hard to say.

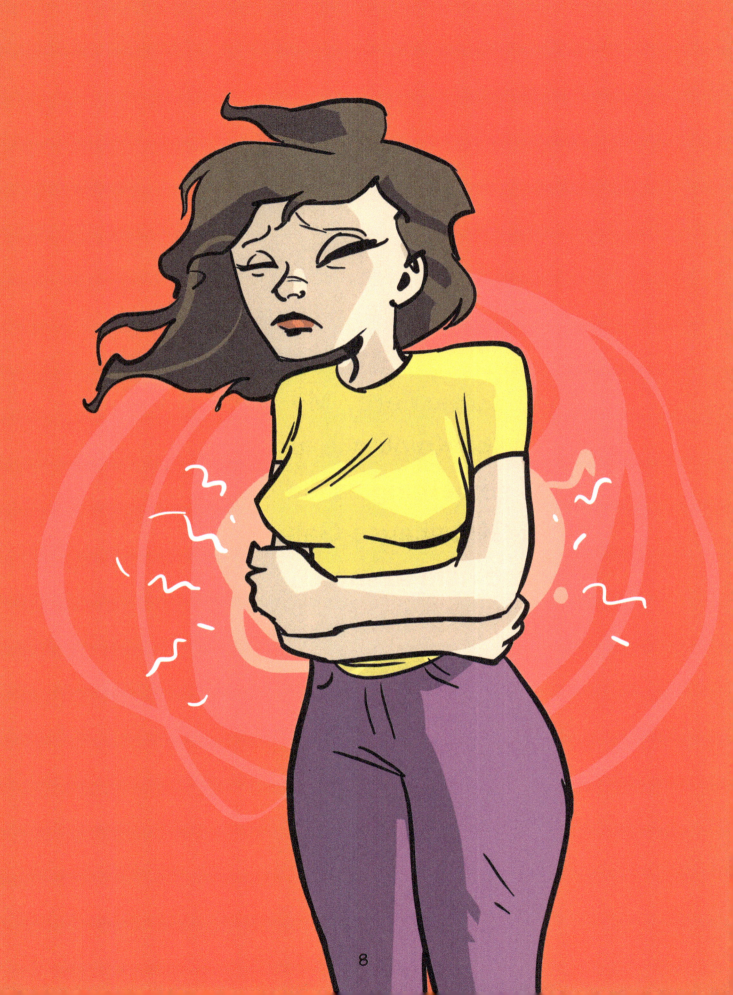

GP means...My Mom's stomach doesn't work. It's paralyzed which is just another way of saying frozen.

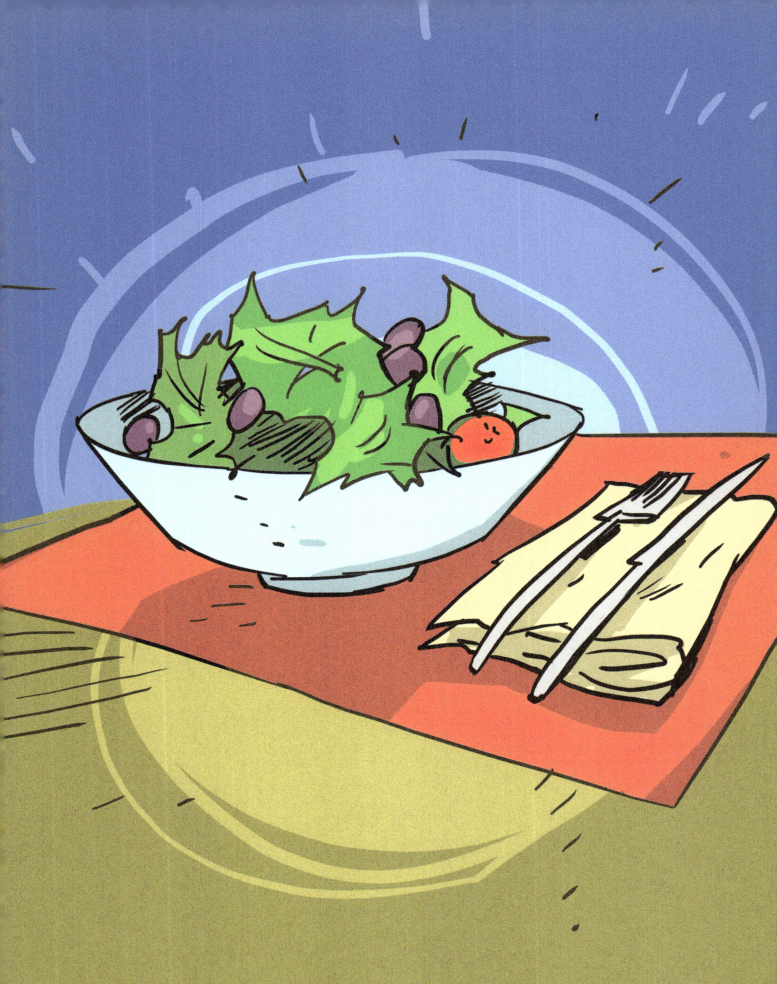

The reason it's her weakness is because it's makes it really hard to get vitamins and energy from the stuff she eats. You know how parents and teachers always tell you to eat your vegetables and eat healthy so you can grow strong? Turns out they are telling the truth because my mom can't eat that stuff and has to take all kind of medicine just to give her the same energy and stuff you would get when you eat a salad.

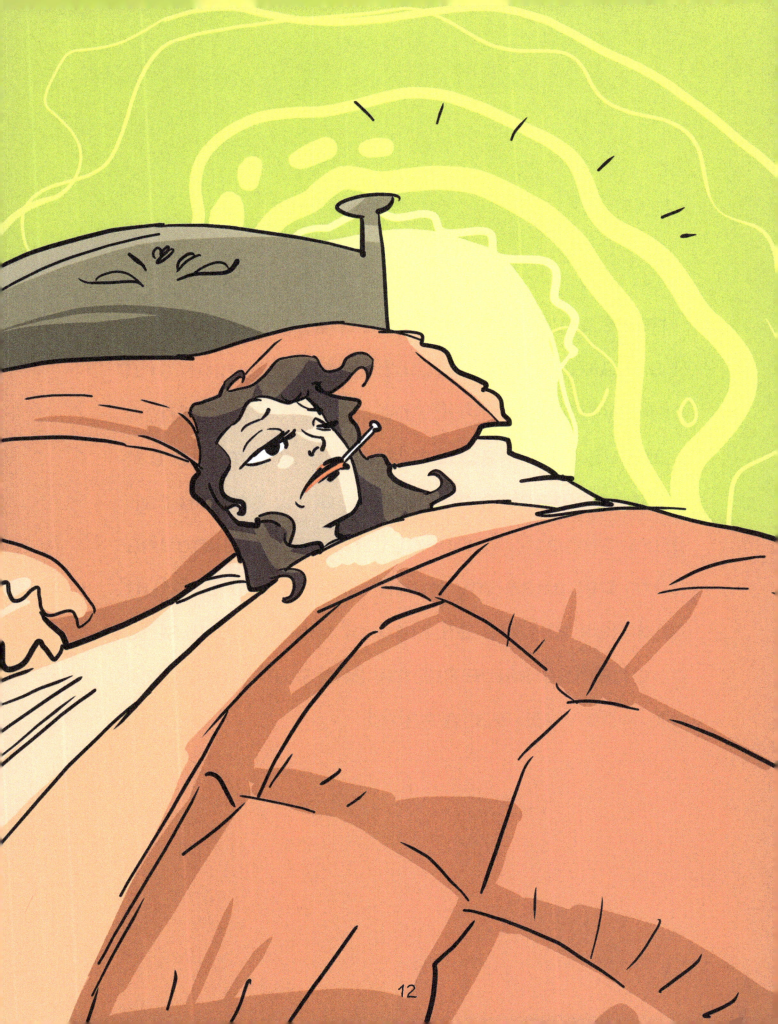

Imagine the worst flu you ever had. The yucky tummy, the achy legs, being tired and just feeling gross. That's what my mom and anyone who has GP feels like almost every day!

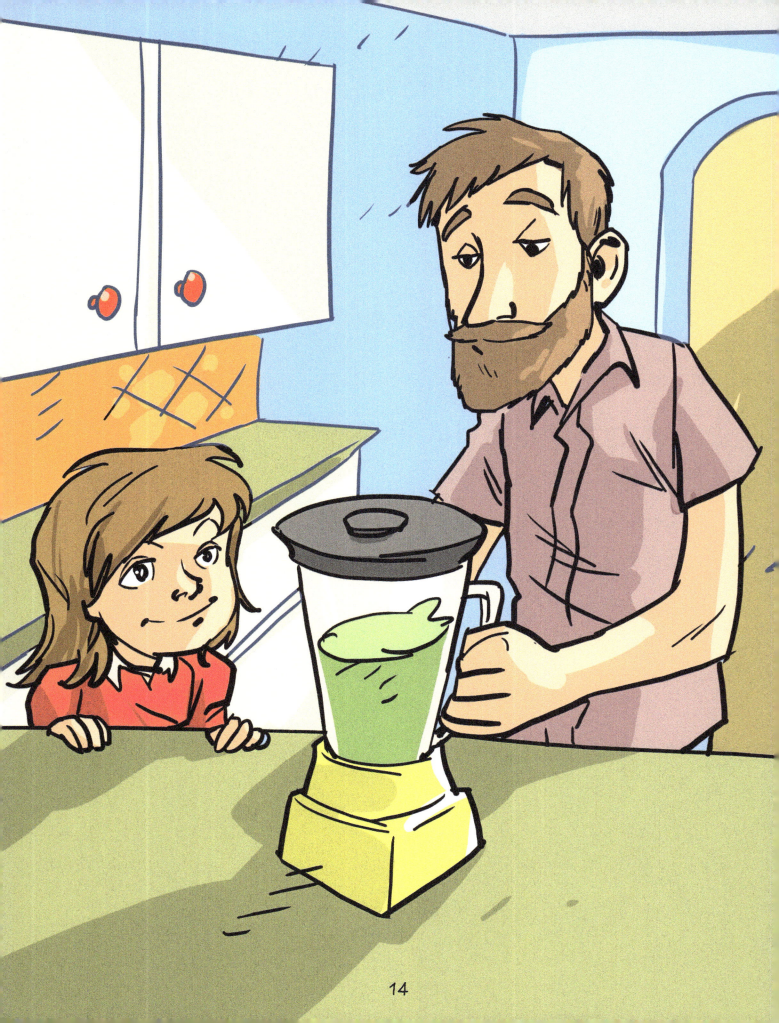

Because of all of this my Mom has a special diet, she has to eat a lot of small meals, a lot of mushy food but she gets to have shakes and stuff a lot at least.

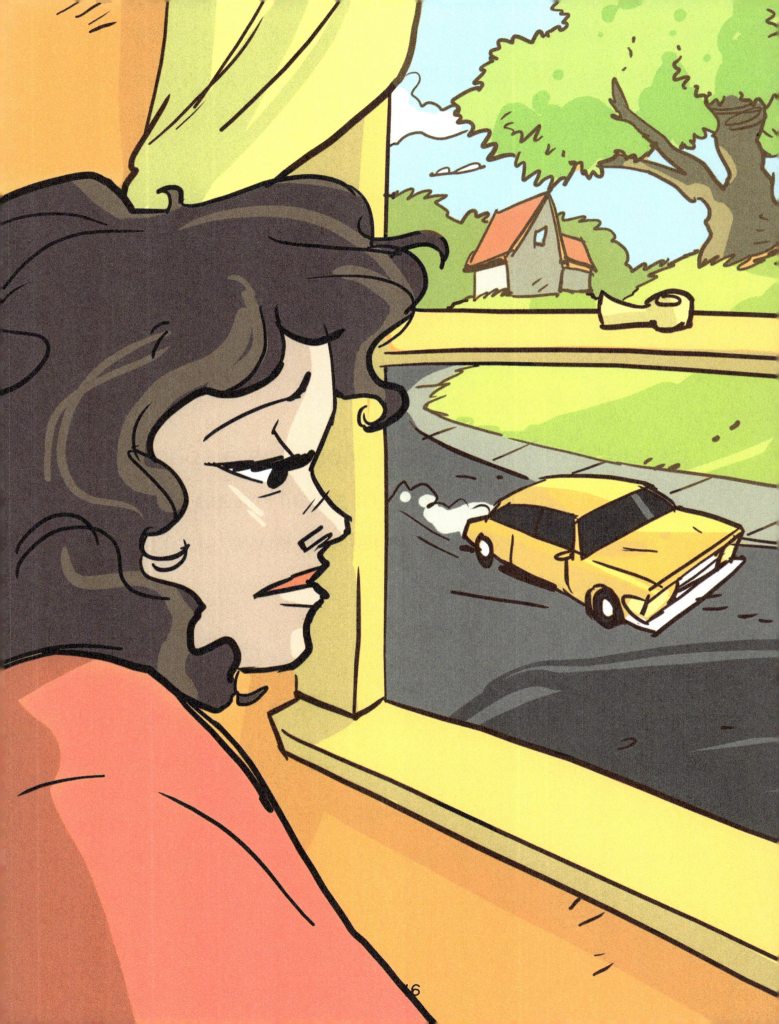

Sometimes because of the GP my Mom just can't do some things. Sometime she misses my games or my sister's dance class. It makes her sad and she says she is sorry a lot, but I always know it's not because she doesn't want to. It's because she doesn't have the energy and is too sick.

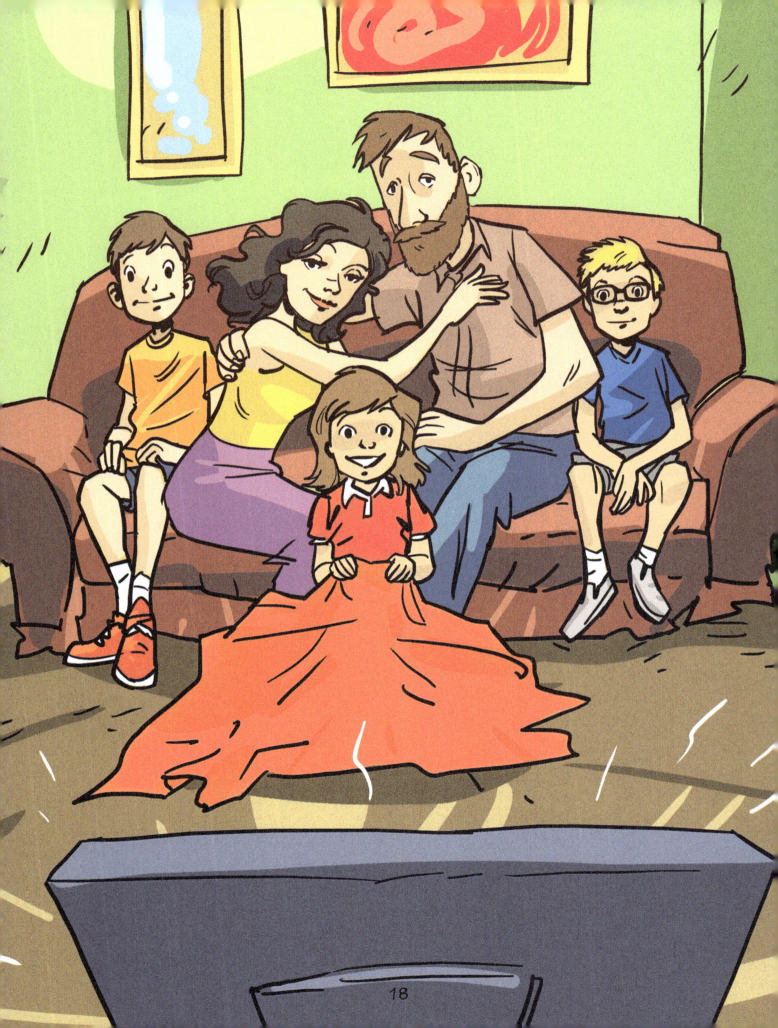

So we make sure when she does feel good and is having a good day we have a lot of fun!

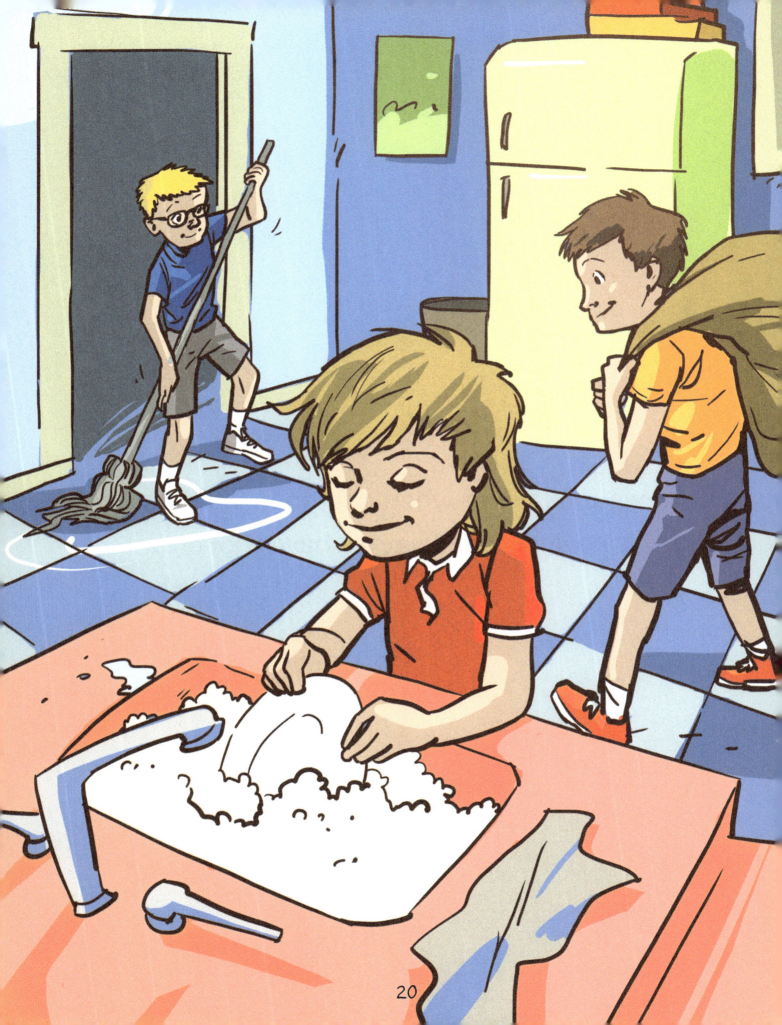

We all try to help around the house so that everything gets done and Mom doesn't have to worry about it. It's a team effort.

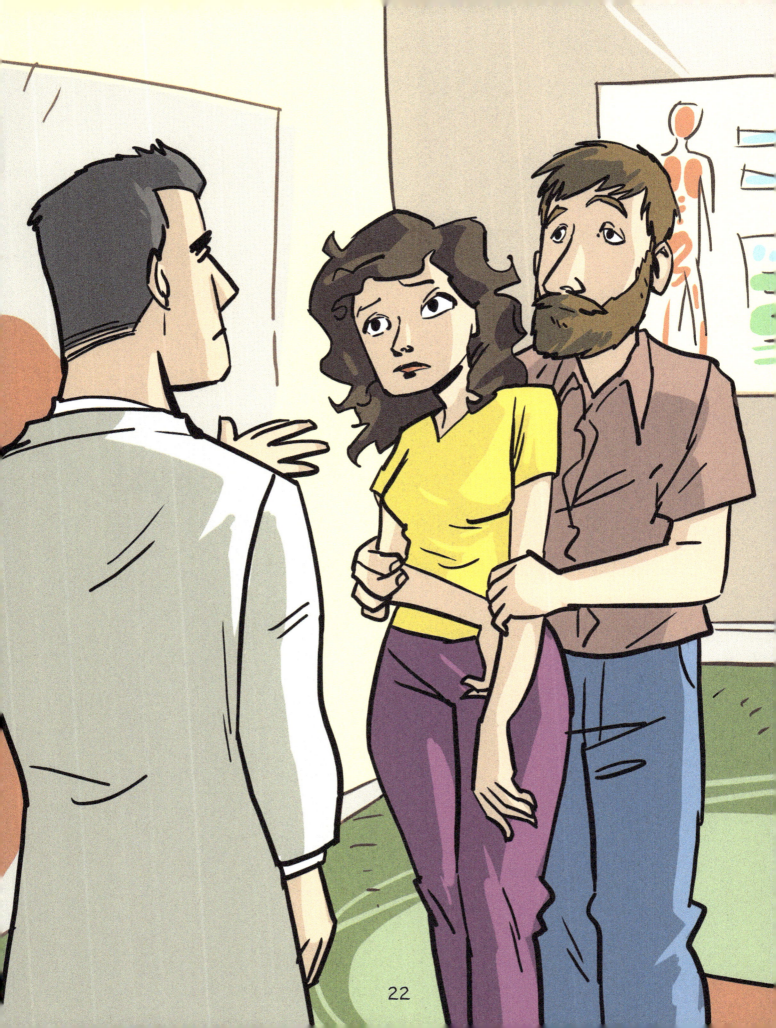

The doctors don't really know how to fix GP, there isn't any magic medicine to make it better.

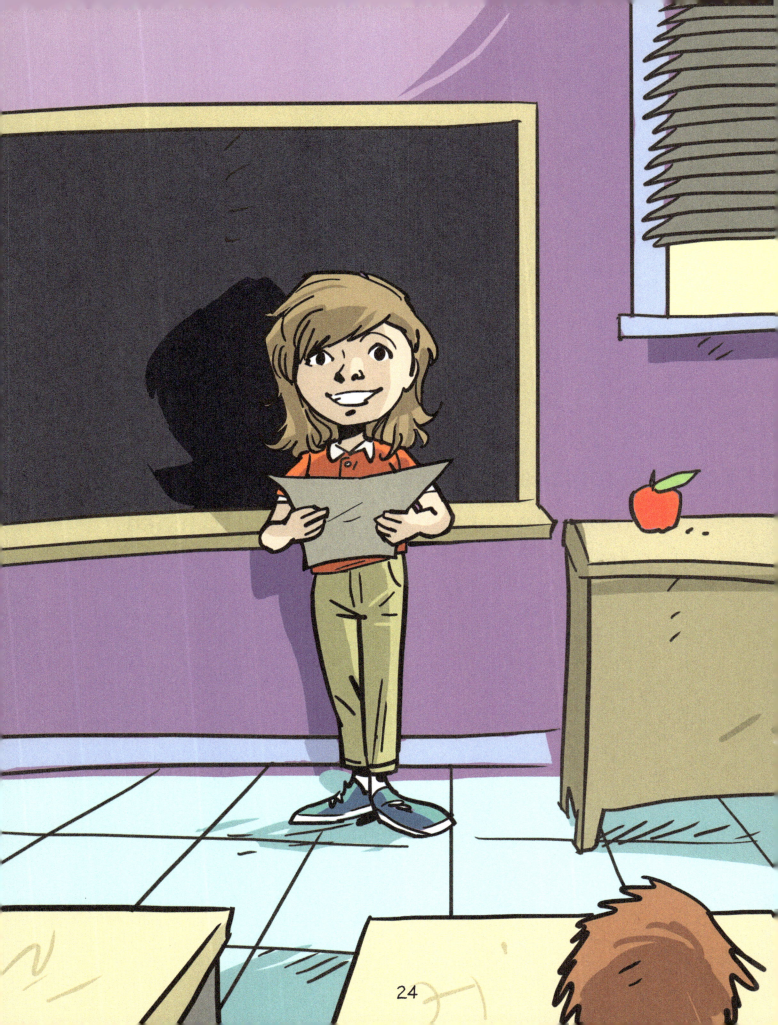

So we have to tell everyone we can about GP so more people want to help, I did a school project about it.

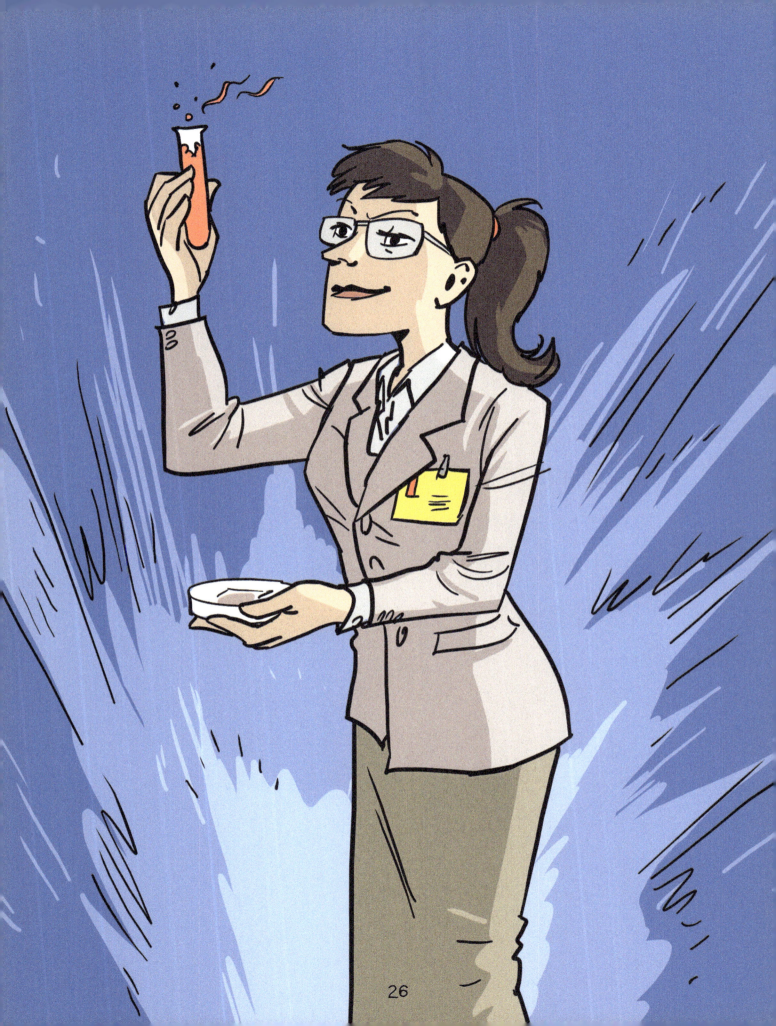

If enough people learn about it, one day scientists will find a way to stop GP forever.

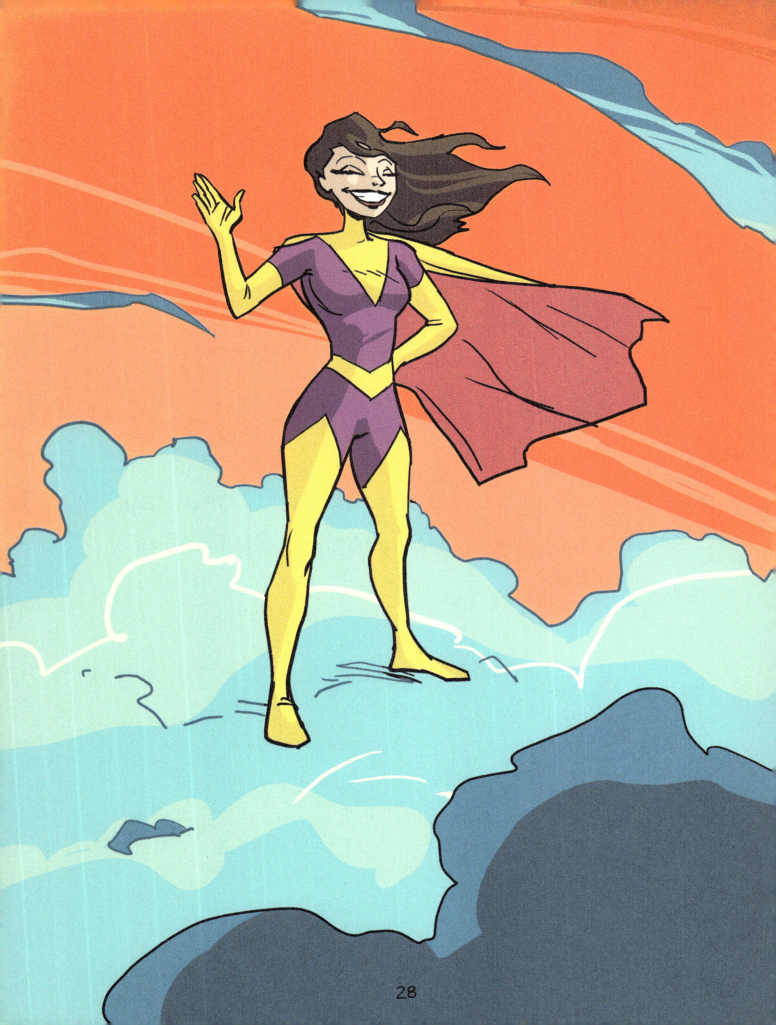

My mom may be sick, but she is still my hero. She is the strongest woman I have ever seen.

CPSIA information can be obtained
at www.ICGtesting.com
Printed in the USA
LVOW05s0851060417
PP12086500001B/6/P